Copyright © 2014 by Mala Wijeweera. PID 602502

ISBN: Softcover 978-1-493-1-4108-1
Ebook 978-1-493-1-4109-8

All rights reserved. No part of this book may be reproduced or transmitted in any form or by any means, electronic or mechanical, including photocopying, recording, or by any information storage and retrieval system, without permission in writing from the copyright owner.

Rev. date: 05/06/2014

To order additional copies of this book, contact:
Xlibris LLC
0-800-056-3182
www.xlibrispublishing.co.uk
Orders@ Xlibrispublishing.co.uk

COSMETIC SURGERY

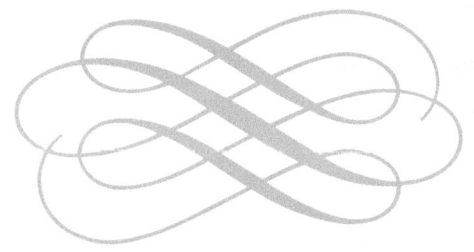

Written by
MALA WIJEWEERA

Acknowledgement

This document is written to get an idea of cosmetic surgery and technical information for medical students and nursing staff in NHS or Private sector in the field of surgery. Written by Mala Wijeweera qualified operating theatre nurse St Georges hospital London 1971.

Contents

Cosmetic-beauty and social acceptance as a necessity 6

Counselling with patient 6

Lipo-sculpture/Lipo-suction/Collagen and skin 7

Vaser lipo surgery 8

Penoplasty 9

Blephroplasty 10

Rhinoplasty 10

Face lift 11

Breast Reduction 12

Breast Implants 12

Hair Transplant 15

Otoplasty 15

Chin implants 16

Abdominoplasty 16

Reversal of Vasectomy 17

Gluteoplasty or Buttock Implants 17

Other operations 18

Testicular Implants 19

Anaesthesia in cosmetic surgery and theatre recovery of patients 19

Cosmetic-beauty and social acceptance as a necessity

Cosmetic surgery is a highly competitive surgical field that needs recognition like any other area of the National Health Service. Throughout history most people have recognized beauty as a key to social acceptance. However, there are many and varied societies and cultures of the world have different ideas of what is Beautiful, although there are some generally accepted standards of beauty such as smooth, unblemished skin, slenderness, shapely figures, large eyes, firm breasts and buttocks etc. The Japanese would bring up young girls feet with care because they consider small and dainty is beautiful.

Counselling with patient

Counselling is necessary before all cosmetic surgery as most patients have no knowledge of procedures involved and therefore they have to be prepared for what may happen and given a clear idea of what to expect to avoid disappointment or shock. The surgeon has a duty to inform the patient of the dangers involved and the possibility that some things may go wrong and that he or she also must cover the legal aspects and obtain the consent of the patient for any procedures. One must point out the risks of disfigurement, disappointment and possible scaring. The patient has to understand that he or she undergoes cosmetic or elective surgery at his or her own risk.

With procedures such as breast implants for example, the surgeon must discuss the dangers of infection if the implant ruptures or the bodies natural defences reject the implant. Haemotoma, bleeding or blood clotting, bruising, swelling and the formation of scar tissue. All have to be considered, as much as the cost of the procedure and the patient ability to pay. These things must be dealt with before admission.

Fear of surgery is another obstacle to be taken in to account and overcome if possible. With local anaesthetic the patient is usually aware of every thing that is happening, this can be quite unnerving and may prefer general anaesthesia.

Lipo-sculpture/Lipo-suction/Collagen and skin

The most common procedure in cosmetic surgery is the removal of excess fat Liposuction from areas of the body where it is prominent. However in a another procedure Lipo-sculpture. The fat is collected from those areas and inserted elsewhere such as the abdomen, hips, thighs, buttock, arms chin, lips and breasts, where it is most needed. Surgeons gradually introduce a solution containing 2%plain xylocaine, 40mls to a 1 liter of sodium chloride, salt, with 1 ampule of 1:1000 adrenaline and a 10mls ampoule of bicarbonate of soda. The Klein solution breaks down the fat in a few minutes inside the body in the areas where liposuction is performed in the subcutaneous layer. Excess fat is extra weight for the body. Fat acts as padding for certain areas of the body and it also has nutritional value as stored fuel for the body, protecting, insulating and stimulating the absorption of nutrional materials, but the body should not have too much surplus fat over and above what is required to maintain health. when a person has too much fat and is over weight, or obese, in appearance it is very embarrassing for both for them and others.

There are different types of fat, such as white fat, yellow fat and greasy, wax like material, in animals, plants, and seeds. The pure fat has no colour, odour or taste. Fat exists in the body as both liquid and solid fatty acids.glycerol provides fuel and energy to the body. There are saturated and unsaturated fats, which are both important and should be included in a properly balanced diet. Unsaturated fat, such as those found in olive oil, vegetable oil, oil based margerine are believed to help to reduce cholesterol levels in the blood. Epidemiological studies in different countries have shown a correlation between fat consumption and breast cancer mortality rates.

The surgeons use long,short,thick,thin and fine cannulas to suck out the fat from various parts of the body in to a bottle,using suction tubes attached to them. the procedure is very common.it can be used in any part of the body,giving instant results of fat removal and a shapelier figure. Most models use cosmetic surgery to improve their career prospects. There is another method of fat removal, using ultrasonic suction with a drip of saline solution going in to the subcutaneous tissues to help to break down the lumps of fatty deposits and smooth out the subcutaneous tissue. This technique is often used as a secondary procedure to the one mentioned above. This process is much gentler on the body than the more aggressive method of lipo suction. The skin is sewn or covered with special dressings and no scars are visible as only very small incisions are made just to get the cannulas inside. Pressure bandages, pads and support garments are used to hold the figure in place during the healing process.

Collagen is a protein substance that changes in case of ageing in lower layer of the dermis angles in bundles of fibers, theseform a pattern of natural creases in the skin. The reticular angular layer is named after Austrian scientist langers lines, cleavage lines of the skin.

When the skin is open to ultra violet rays or direct sunlight more than required skin is prone to skin cancer. Skin sags and buckle and folds and creases although sunlight increases the production of melanin that gives pigment colour to the skin and protect the skin from any damage and helps to produce vitamin D the skin looses the water. The molecules linked with long chains. The connective tissue that act as a cushion to organs takes place with age and slow down sebaceous glands and sweat glands.

The epidermis is the outer layer of the skin. Some have freckles, moles, birth marks.some are benign and some are malignant, skin is a special sense receptor with nerve endings scattered through out the body like a network. feeling of heat, cold, pain,touch and pressure can be regulated through the skin.

The surgeons use local and general anaesthetics or intravenous sedation or pseudo-analgesia. There is always tissue trauma and shock associated with operative procedures and discomfort will disappear after short time. Allergic reactions, skin rashes are very common, exposed to extreme heat or cold will kill the tissues and become gangrenous.

Vaser lipo surgery

The vaser machine is used to infiltrate0.9% sodium chloride, bicarbonate of sodium10mls and 40mls of xylocaine and 1 ampoule of adrenaline 1:1000 for each liter of saline. Each area of the body is controlled by time.

Bodylift-lipo surgery. This procedure is done as a secondary treatment for liposuction using a bodylift machine and necessary equipment. One has to observe controlled energy output to each area of the body. Micro air lipo suction this is a comfortable machine operated procedure for liposuction that gives good results and it is safe for the patient.

Penoplasty

Through out the human history, men have wanted to be macho and impress women with their sexual prowes. In primitive cultures, there is plenty of evidence of the use of a form of traction, attaching weights to the penis to lengthen it and increase its girth to satisfy the women and themselves, during sexual intercourse. Presumbably they believed that these techniques would strengthen and prolong the erection, thus improving their ability to perform.most poets and writers have used rubber bands, strings, caps, moulds, and heavy keys and even stones to put weight on to the penis to stretch the unfortunate organ.

These methods were not known to many people as it was a well kept secret. Hereditary and hormonal growth and development and cultural factors are related to this problem. There are many causes of physiological, psychological and emotional aspects to this problem in men the medical profession has ignored this aspect in human beings. They carried a feeling of impotence due to fatigue, illness, stress, anxiety and some states of marital problems. Some suffered Alcoholism depressing the central nervous system, preventing sexual satisfaction in the woman. Testicular dysfunction is another obstruction in the hormone levels in the blood of the male organs. These days men tend to prefer plastic surgery to increase the length of their manhood, this operation is quite common among men, particularly in the affluent countries of the western world today. Most men who undergo this procedure like the instant increase in the length of their penis.

However no doubt many are disappointed by the less spectacular result when the improvement does not quite measure up to their expectations. The surgeons pay more attention to the psychological needs of the partners through counselling. Doctors use medical methods while sex therapist use other techniques to help overcome these problems as more and more marriages are coming to an end.some become drug addicts,heavy smokers and even attempt suicide because they feel inadequate. The increase in sexual crime, violence, prostitution, the spread of Aids and other sexually transmitted diseases have all been link to these problems. The surgeons use a scientific approach, severing the suspensory ligament to increase the length of the penis. This is accomplished by making a small incision just above the penis, raising a flap of skin giving access to the suspensory ligament taking care not to damage the surrounding veins,nerve fibers blood vessels ect, allowing the penis to hang free,giving the appearance of greater length. To increase the thickness of the penis. Fat is removed from elsewhere and inject under the skin A special solution designed for the purpose. This is a simple procedure that can be performed under a local or general anaesthetic according to the patients preference. Most men have been satisfied with the result.

Blephroplasty

Blephroplasty is a very simple operation, it can be done under general or local anaesthesia or with laser surgery. The fatty tissues around the eyes are removed from the upper and lower eyelids. The surgeons make a very fine incision midway between the eyebrow and the eye lashes and also correct the canthus of the eye. The surgeons use a very fine bipolar diathermy to cauterise the blood vessels. There is upper and lower blephroplasty. The patient is very safe and looks very good. Most people look at the eyes for beauty and appearance. Cold compress, eye ointment and special dressings are used to heal the wounds around.

Rhinoplasty

The nose is the centre of attraction in all human beings. Noses come in an amazing variety of shapes and sizes and can often reveal a great deal about a persons ethnic origins. For example, there is the roman nose, The aquiline, eagle nose, bulbous nose, often though not always indicative of a heavy drinker and the negroid nose which tends to be flatter and broader than the Caucasian varieties. The main reason for this diversity of nasal dimensions is the fact that most humans fall in to one of four basic physiological groups, indo- European, mongoloid, negroid and oriental. Some people for one reason or another are unhappy with the shape and size of their nose and those who can afford it choose cosmetic or reconstructive surgery to correct what they perceive to be defect. There are also medical conditions which may require the services of plastic surgeons such as deviated septum, which can cause difficulties with breathing and possibly speech impediments, which can be corrected surgically. Many people select to have their noses altered simply to improve their appearances because they feel that it is too big, too small, or misshape in some way that makes them less attractive than might otherwise be, others choose cosmetic or reconstructive surgery because of respiratory difficulties or accidental injury or disfigurement due to disease or to try to recover the sense of smell which is connected to taste. Some have problems to do with congestion of sinuses. Surgeons reconstruct the nose by removing, or reshaping pieces of cartilage and bone. Once the problem is corrected the nose is supported with plaster of paris or splints with special dressings to hold every thing in place while the wounds heal. Most people are quite pleased with the results.

Face lift

Excessive facial lines, jowls droopiness the neck can be corrected by laser surgery or with incision within the hairline at the temples, smoothing out ridges and wrinkles. Surgeons do a full face and neck lift to women, men like a lift from the forehead as it does not interfere with the shaving skin. Facial skin is cut in to shape by dissecting and separating the facial skin from the subcutaneous tissue down to the chin and lifting up the facial muscles with stitches, paying careful attention to facial nerves, haemoraging and tissue damage. Excess skin is cut off in shape behind the ears and sewn up with fine stitches or staples and drains are used to drain the haemotoma. The wounds are dressed with cotton wool and tight bandages to hold the skin in place while they heal. The dissection and infiltration to skin and tissues take a long time as great care has to be taken not to disfigure the patient. The face lifts done by specialist surgeons have good results and the patients look beautiful and it is mostly skin lift. So, beauty really is, skin deep. It is challenging for women to look beautiful and graceful in old age. In wisdom of health. It is revolutionary one has to intergrate with the new knowledge for women about anti-ageing looks for the face, body and spirit in order to feel gorgeous in health and body, one must follow simple exercises, nutrition supplements and skin care in rejuvenating with cosmetic surgery. In biological ageing beauty sleep and stress control are important.

Wrinkles and sagging skin depends on the life style one leads. For instance excessive alcohol, smoking, dehydrates the skin, also exposure to direct and excessive sunlight, pollution of air, excessive weight loss results in skin sagging. Stretching, dryness of skin, wrinkles, jowls and tiredness because of the lack of oxygen degenerates the skin. Collagen fibre and elastin support the skin. Make-up inspires women. Age spots, wrinkles, fine lines, redness can be corrected. Mini face lift " S" lift. The surgeons excise the skin around the ears, pulls up the skin, tightens the mascular poneurotic facia fibrous tissue and sling muscle which covers the jaw line, removing the excess skin also known as the skin lift.

Breast Reduction

Breast reduction for oversized and misshapen breasts due to cancer operations etc. are very uncomfortable and embarrassing for most women. They come for breast reduction to have them made smaller, firmer, shapely and more evenly balanced. Many women do not realize that it is quite normal to have one breast slightly larger than the other, because they imagin that they look lopsided.

The excess fatty tissues are removed and carefully weighed and measured. The surgeons make an incision around the areoles and the nipples and are carefully repositioned. Dressings are used to protect the wounds and hold them in place while they heal. As it is a major procedure it is available in nhs as well as in private practice. The surgeons make a left lateral, right lateral, medial and central excisions giving consideration to the pedicles of the breasts of the patients.

Breast Implants

Breast augmentation or mammary implants vary in size and texture according to the products used and the patients preference. There are micro-cell, silicone gel and various other fillings for the prosthetics. The patient must be fully informed of the risks involved and possible complications of placing foreign bodies in to the chest wall. Loss of sensation nerve damage capsular contractions due to formation of fibrous tissues around the implants are all risks that must be considered by the patient before undergoing surgery. Sometimes skin cells can break down due to ageing, infection, accidents and haemotoma or displacement which can cause wrinkles and make patients very embarrassed and uncomfortable. Some prosthesis have been known to leak or cause other complications, such as the formation of hard lumps, scars, and pain. Calcium deposits can form around the implants Ruptured implants must be removed and replaced immediately. Adequate sized surgical pockets must be created to avoid tissue irritation, swelling, pain, tederness, fever or sarcoma formation due to infection. These conditions will delay the healing process. Having periods during operations must be considered as strands from during menstruation making dissection difficult for surgeons. All the medical conditions must be attendend to by the surgeons.

Horizontal creases, lines below the breasts must be observed. A pocket is tunnelled behind the breast, but in front of the chest muscle. It is important to measure the correct volume before dissection of the pocket in the chest wall and major pectoral muscle not disturbing the mammary glands and nerves. Surgical procedures demands the correct position or plane of dissection for the volume of the implants and strict aseptic techniques to avoid the risk of infection. The surgeons must take care not to puncture the prosthesis and to wash them in a special solution before implanting them in to the patient as some of them are oily and are made from soya bean oil, which are bio-compatible with breasts fatty tissues and dietary fats according to medical grades triglycerides. Surgeons make a 4cm incision as breast tissues are very thin and sensitive. Implants are placed sub glandular or sub pectoral or making axillary approach or peri- areole or trans aereole or sub mammary incision for cosmetic or reconstructive surgery or to correct congenital deformities. Once the prostheses is placed in the breast pocket or cavity, after checking the haemotoma, the incision is closed using fine sutures and dressings are applied and a bra, plaster or bandages are used to hold the prosthesis in place while the wounds heal.

Trilucent implants based on soya bean oil have had adverse effect on osmotic pressure in many patients apart from capsular obstruction and contraction due to formation of fibrous tissues surrounding the implants, therefore surgeons have been using water and sugar based (hydrogel) implants instead as breast prosthesis of patients. Saline filled mammary implants are also in use as saline is isotonic with blood plasma. Perforations can occur due to external compression and internal haemotoma. Silicone implants have been damaged internally on many occasions and have had be removed surgically, both in national health and private sector in the past. There was an increasing demand for trilucent and cloverleaf implants,rather than silicone or gel-filled with which there have been some problems. With the texture, profile and shape. Trilucent implants have been taken off the market because it is a contributing factor cancer. We have removed thousands of such implants from patients in the past in the operating theatres.

Most women in the United kingdom and America use this procedure. It is particularly popular with models and others, page three girls,bay watch beauties,glamour models,fashion models and others who wish to improve their cleavage. Men wishing to have sex change or "gender reassignment"also come in for breast implants instead of or as well as hormone replacement therapy. In United Kingdom National Health Service plastic surgeons only perform these procedures in special cases, such as to correct congenital or hereditary deformities, accidental disfigurement or cancer patients who require extensive reconstructive surgery.

There is an increasing demand for breast augmentation to improve employment, financial and marital prospects to offer the older woman the illusion of looking and feeling younger, but it cannot halt or even slow down the natural ageing process, nor can it cure mental illness or depression or obsession with ones who physical appearance, however it may restore confidence for someone who has elected to have some disfigurement corrected, other than that it is no more than vanity.they may think they look and possibly even feel younger, but they are not really, they deceive only themselves.

Cosmetic surgeons correct physical disfigurements and deformities to help their patients regain lost confidence, self-esteem and acceptance in society and in business. Some people however elected to have cosmetic surgery to improve their appearance and enhance their career and marital prospects.

Hair Transplant.

Hair transplant usually involve the careful removal of pieces of skin (where healthy follicles are present) from the back of the scalp or the sides, to the areas where they are needed to replace the lost hair. Most people who have had this treatment are generally very satisfied with the results. This technique is most commonly used as a cure for hair loss or male pattern baldness as it is more commonly known, however it is not only men who suffer from hair loss, some women also experience this problem. The treatment involves transplanting healthy roots of hair from one area of the scalp to where they are needed to replace lost hairs using a local anaesthetic to reduce the blood loss and pain and allow the surgeon to make tiny incisions and insert metal plugs in to the sub-dermal layers of the scalp to anchor the roots in place,where after afew weeks they begin to grow normally again.

Self-esteem is very important to most people these days and some women have been known to use this method to transplant hair roots in the pubic areas.

Otoplasty

Otoplasty is to do with the ears and usually means pinning them back by removing part of the cartilage from behind the ear and carefully sewing the ear in to this new position, the results of which are usually very satisfying to the patient.

Removal of tattoos,marks and moles also commonly requested procedures. Some of the methods used include dermal abration and skin grafts. Plastic surgeons are called upon to perform a remarkable variety of other procedures too. For example fat insertion (re-alocation) silicone implants for the scrotum,calves. buttocks, etc. Many patients require plastic surgery to repair damage done to them through no fault of their own or deformities, disfigurements and defects caused by congenital conditions, accidental injury, land mines, cancer, burns, birthmarks, cleft palates, abnormalities of the genital organs, web fingers, and toes, flabby stomachs and many other problems whether real or perceived.

Chin implants

These operations are being performed to give greater definition and firmness to the chin. An incision is made between the gum and the lower lip and the implant is inserted, then the skin and soft subcutaneous tissues are sewn back. Skin grafts are made and used for upper and lower lip augmentations. Collagen injection is another technique used for lip enhancement. Supplies of human skin subcutaneous tissues and collagen have been collected by live tissue banks in theUnited States of America and the Uniliver Research Laboratories in the United Kingdom.

Abdominoplasty.

The operation is performed by cosmetic surgeons to reduce the over hanging, Bulging. Abdominal tissues. One must consider the structures of the abdomen and incision by marking the the skin with heavy muscles in front and sides. The diaphragm separates the lower part of the chest. The upper abdomen and the lower abdomen. The pelvic area of the body, peritoneum lining, the abdominal wall protects the internal organs of the body. In reconstruction of the abdomen the surgeons make a transverse incision and remove the excess bulging abdominal tissues and make un shapely area shapely. They also use lipo suction technique to reduce the fat from the tissues. Strong sutures are being used with round bodied needles to keep the area strong and firm taking care of undue pressure on the abdomen as it affects the breathing and internal organs of the body. In re-adjusting the umbilicus measurements are being taken from the sides and the lower part of the abdomen to re-position the umbilicus. Some surgeons use artistic incisions in the lower abdominal area to avoid dog ears on the sides. It is important to wash out the wounds with anti- biotic solution prior to closure of the wounds to avoid seroma forming after the operation. Abdominal supports are being used after the operation and dressings with less discomfort. Positioning of patients is also important in this operation while operating and after the operation.

Reversal of Vasectomy

Vasectomy, a sterilization system for men to block the spermatosa in testicles by excising the vas deferens, a section of the ducts that transport the sperm from testes is available on the National Health Services to patients who for various reasons do not wish to have children. However some patients decide to have the procedure reversed. In reversal procedure cosmetic surgeons use microsurgery techniques to look carefully in to the vas deferens and both sides of the severed ducts are picked up cleaned, dilated and irrigated to clear the passage and they are sewn back together again with very fine eye sutures of nylon or prolene. Once he has recovered the patients should be able to reproduce normally, assuming that he was able to reproduce before having the vasectomy!

Gluteoplasty or Buttock Implants.

The two gluteal muscles are situated behind the hip covered with flesh and are strong giving posture and support to the spinal column and make a seat to the human body. The surgeon Mr. Shiva Dayal Singh(fellow of the college of surgeons Edinburgh/England)who performs the operations with the patient positioned in prone position. The surgeon make a subcutaneous bi-section and use a hockey stick spatula dissector to make space for the silicone shapely implants. Most implants are soaked in antibioti IV saline lotion or powder prior to insertion or introduction. The antibiotic in the IV saline drip to reduce the risk of infection and tissue damage or further complications to the implant area. The silicone implants are placed under the Gluteus Maximus and rest on top of the gluteus medius on both sides, giving attention to the sciatic nerve, the longest and strongest4/5cm in breadth in the sacral plexus inside the pelvis. Gluteoplasty or buttock implants or buttock up lifts are very common and fashion-conscious surgery. Modern trends are to have rounded buttocks and narrow waistline. Fat insertions to depress areas of the buttocks has been very successful surgery. The idea of getting the excess skin in the buttock up lifted or removed or filled with fat are a fashion. There are men and women who come for this operation.

Other operations.

Fat Transfer. Most surgeons gather the fat autologus process for a longer life. Areas of body recontouring and inserting-fat in to depressed areas, buttocks, thighs, knees, face, neck, chin, arms, waist, abdomen and breasts. There is also liposuction or liposculpture for the same areas of the body like in abdominoplasty. Ultrasonic liposuction probes dissolves fat, sucking it out of the body The latest micro cannulas are used by surgeons. Vaser liposuction gives patients good results.

Endoscopic brow lift. The type of surgery is similar to key hole sub periosteal lift surgery. The surgeons uses an endoscope and endoscopic scissors to cut and long instruments to sew up the incisions and washout. Chemical skin peels. These types of peels are been used on the face with chemicals and alphahydroxy aids.

Derma Abrasion. The surgeons use derma abrasion instruments for the upper lips and face. Collagen injection. The surgeon injects the forehead and wrinkled areas of the face. Botox, Gortex or soft form is used for patient to enhance the lips and autologus fat as fillers for reshaping and do laser resurfacing. Calf implants. Some men and women enjoy having good legs. Silicone implants of various sizes are placed in the calves of legs. The surgeons make a small incision at the back of the legs, in the prone position paying attention to the lateral popliteal nerve and other structures. The surgeons use a hockey stick instrument and spatula to make a tunnel to receive the implant.

Arm lift Women like to get rid of excessive fat, tissues and skin near the armpits. The surgeons excise the tissue and sews up the incision or use liposuction inside upper armpits. Gynaecomastia. To get rid of the excess fat and tissue from the chest in men. Lipo suction is some time used. In major cases the excess tissue around the nipple is taken out. Labial Reduction. This operation is very common and popular amongst women. Labia minora is also called labia plasty. The excess skin is excised and the hanging skin reduced. Nipple Lift. Both men and women can have nipple correction. Inverted nipples are uplifted and crrected by surgeons.

Thigh Lift. Many women have thigh operations to get rid of the excess tissue and skin between the upper thigh and inner areas. Cheek Implants.

Silicone cheek implants up lift the facial cheeks. The operation is done from inside the cheek.

ChinImplants. The operation is done with silicone implants from inside the jaw.

Breast Implants. In recent times breast up lifts are performed by making the incision below the nipple making a vertical incision. AdamsApple. This operation is performed by surgeons with the patients neck carefully exposed and a small incision is made in the neck and the Adams apple is shaved. The jaw is also opened with a small incision from inside. The chin bone is burred from inside and sewn by the surgeon.

Testicular Implants

Men have silicone testicular implants in the tesicles which have been damaged by environment conditions or congenital problems. This is a successful operation.

Laser Liposuction. This procedure is done by the use of a laser light (beam) introduced to the subcutaneous tissue with controlled energy out put and infiltration to areas of the body.

Anaesthesia in cosmetic surgery and theatre recovery of patients

It is vitally important to observe procedure when administering anaesthetic drugs, gases and agents and the responses of individuals during surgical procedures. Skin is a very sensitive organ which covers and protects the underlying tissue from the environment. Micro-organisms such as bacteria and viruses and other potentially harmful substances. The epidermis(outer layer of the skin)when exposed to ultraviolet rays can be irritated and damaged(which can lead to melanoma or skin cancer). The dermis, the deeper layer consist of capillaries, nerves, nerve endings, lymph, melanin, epithelial cells, sweat glands, oil glands and hair follicles, connective tissue to the sensory organs of the outer layer that give us sensivity to touch, pressure, heat, cold, pain, injury etc.

Between the epidermis and the dermis is an intermediate, granular layer of fat transparent cells. Before any anaesthesia can be administered those responsible must be aware of any potential problems that may occur due to such things as the patients weight, acardiac problems, metabolic disorders or hereditary traits that may cause an allergic or adverse reaction to the anaesthetic drugs being used also any possible reaction to bio-chemicals or drugs present in the patients blood and muscle fibers, such as calcium, potassium, prophylactic support drugs, muscle relaxants, etc. It is very important to monitor all these factors during surgical procedures. Tubular blockages, peripheral perfusions are also important to avoid tachycardia, bradycardia, scoline, apnoea an to avoid secondary cardiac arrest after correction of respiratory out put, cardiac compression and ventilation.

Post operative anaesthesia, post operative analgesia and reversing stages of anaesthesia of unconscious patients are the responsibilities of the anesthetist. The cardiovascular, respiratory and central nervous systems are the areas to watch when avoiding upper respiratory tract obstruction. Most anesthetists ignore the response in the cosmetic surgery as it is easier to work on the visible areas of the skin than inside the body and the internal organs. It is the same with the local anaesthetic, intravenous infusion and sedative analgesia.

Theatre recovery of patients. This area is the most important part of the surgical work in cosmetic surgery. Patients come to recovery with different operative procedures and dressings over areas operated. The patient has to be looked after with care by the nurse, conscious, semi-conscious patients need four to five liters of oxygen. Patients need to be made comfortable and warm and monitored, observed with their blood pressure respiration, dressings, drains, that are applied by the surgeons. Post operative analgesia and the administration of fluids must be also done. The nurse needs to speak to the patient about the operation and also pain relief. Any drains attached to the patients wounds must be checked, dressings must be intact. The patient must be fully conscious before going back to the ward. Occasionally the wounds may bleed and hematoma results. These conditions must be reported to the surgeons and anesthetists. The nurse need to see the vital signs of movement of the limbs or jaws in face lifts as well as the colour of the patient in breathing as respiration is important in post operative care.

Consultants

Mr. Bastra	Mr. Kurzer
Mr. Leborne	Mr. Kark
Mr. Jaya Prakash	Mr. Gadir
Mr. Singh	Mr. Stanek
Mr. Roberto Viel	Dr. Obiekwe
Mr. Mauritzio Viel	Mr. Ashby
Mr. Nathan	Mr. Belsham
Mr. Alexandrides	Mr. Latimer Sayer
Mr. S. Khan	Mr. Fratti
Mr. U. Khan	Mr. Davies
Ms. Tatari	Dr. Moustafa
Mr. Chandarasak	Dr. Leader
Mr. Kraema	Dr. Silva
Mr. Aslam	Dr. Saunders
Miss Hazarica	Dr. Chandra
Mr. Percival	Dr. Renna
Miss. Katrina	Dr. King
Mr. Albasri	Dr. Irvine
Mr. Erian	Dr. Samad
Ms. Gill	Dr. Tatari
Mr. Rosen	Dr. Kotak
Mr. Daniel	Dr. Ambrozova
Mr. Ghatak	Dr. Vicary
Mr. Aurakzai	Dr. Cohen
Mr. Iregbulum	Mr. Horn
Dr. Chout	Mr. Marcellino
Mr. Mitra	Mr. Ossie Fernando
Mr. Skanderoiz	Mr Raja Jayaweera
Mr. Agravel	Mr Laws
Mr. Joffley	Mr. Bailey
Mr. Jaward	Dr. Valli Ratnam
Mr. Younis	Dr. Chang

List of hospitals I have worked in UK:

1. University College Hospital
2. Royal Free Hospital
3. Whittington Hospital
4. Highgate Private Hospital
5. Park View Clinic Hospital
6. London Private Hospital
7. Royal Northern Hospital
8. St. Bartholomews Hospital
9. Barnet General Hospital
10. Royal ENT Hospital
11. Cane Hill Hospital
12. Dartford Green Hospital Kent
13. Carshalton Beaches Childrens' Hospital
14. Harley Street Clinic Hospital
15. Humana Hospital
16. Cromwel Hospital
17. Portland Hospital
18. Old Court Hospital
19. Hammersmith Hospital
20. Greenwich Hospital
21. St. Mary's Hospital
22. Nightingale Hospital
23. Mariestopes Clinic Hospital
24. Princess Grace Hospital
25. London Clinic Hospital
26. Heather Green Hospital
27. Frien Barnet Hospital
28. Manor House Hospital
29. Mr. Veils Clinic Hospital
30. Chelsea Hospital
31. British Hernia Clinic Hospital
32. Middlesex Hospital
33. Welbeck Hospital
34. Transform Medical Group Hospitals
35. Dr. Silva's Clinic Perfect Image Hospital
36. Worked in old people's homes
37. Worked as special nurse
38. Worked as escort nurse
39. Worked as agency nurse
40. Worked in general and in cosmetic surgery as E grade nurse

www.ingramcontent.com/pod-product-compliance
Lightning Source LLC
Chambersburg PA
CBHW050438180526
45159CB00006B/2582